# Alkaline Diet

# Recipe Book:

# Alkaline Diet Recipes For Weight Loss, Health and Wellness

By

Valerie Alston

# Table of Contents

Alkaline Diet Recipe Book: Alkaline Diet Recipes For Weight Loss, Health and Wellness

By Valerie Alston

# Introduction

The common foods that people usually eat release either alkaline base or acid into the blood after they pass the digestion process. Foods such as meat, fish, poultry, grains, shellfish, salt, milk and cheese produce acid. Overconsumption of acid releasing foods can cause the body to become over acidic and dispossess of its minerals. In the long run, people who failed to balance their diet with essential alkaline foods may become apt to develop chronic diseases and gain weight.

The alkaline diet or alkaline ash as it is also known is basing its assumption that eating an alkaline rich diet can take off extra pounds and improve one's health. Accordingly, the alkaline diet supports the utilization of completely unprocessed foods. However, people who want to adopt the diet to their daily food planning must be aware that some of the known healthy foods such as legumes, beans and other essential fats may be excluded.

This book has various alkaline diet recipes which will help you to follow the diet.

# Chapter 1. The Foods to Include in Alkaline Diet

Eating fruits and vegetables have to be increased to nine servings per day at least. The diet must be more on root vegetables as well as tubers such as turnips, carrots and beets. Additionally, include tomatoes, avocadoes, lime, bananas, grapefruit and coconut. Whole grains may also be included, but not wheat. Also, include millet, quinoa and buckwheat.

The other foods that can be included in the diet are seeds, nuts and tofu. One can also consider several alkaline rich legumes including lentils and lima beans. If you opt to use oils, choose flax, olive, sesame, coconut and pumpkin.

# Chapter 2. Alkaline Diet Tips

1. Consume more on vegetarian foods because they contain the most alkaline.

2. Prefer whole grains instead of processed foods. Whole grains have greater nutritional content and retain fiber that regulates glucose release, which help in balancing the blood sugar.

3. Several foods that taste acidic such as lime, lemon and grapefruit are turned alkaline when digested, which becomes less burdensome on the digestive process.

4. Cola and coffee are acidic foods, while foods that have the most alkaline are fruits and vegetables such as grapefruit, dates, figs, lime, lemon, artichoke, beetroot, broccoli, asparagus, cauliflower, kale, watercress and spinach.

5. Several alkaline foods have water containing vitamins and minerals that are rather absorbed easily than that of plain bottled water, which allows the body to hydrate from food, not simply from the water we drink.

# Chapter 3. Why Alkaline Diet is Good for Your Health

1. The alkaline diet improves digestion; lessen the flatulence and the bloating of abdomen.

2. The diet improves the skin tone. The nuts, seeds and their oil have great amount of essential fats that made up the skin's matrix.

3. The alkaline diet helps to have better memory, concentration and focus because the blood sugar levels are being regulated over a long while.

4. The diet improves your tendency to be happy. Most of the grains are satisfying the serotin receptors in our gut that helps in elevating the mood.

5. Alkaline diet improves energy levels. Slow-release carbohydrates that help in keeping the blood sugar balance characterize the alkaline foods.

# Chapter 4. Alkaline Diet Food Guidelines

The best way in balancing acid-forming and alkaline-forming foods, when a person is consuming fish, meat or chicken is by following the eighty-twenty rule. The person should get plenty of vegetables that are served with grains as base, and having protein perched right on the top. The diet will ensure the person that majority of his/her meal is alkaline and not sacrificing the foods they enjoy.

**The alkaline-forming foods include:**

a) Fennel, watercress, celery, asparagus and cauliflower

b) Spinach, parsley, rocket, kelp and coriander

c) Garlic, ginger, onion and beetroot

d) Pumpkin, sunflower and sesame seeds

e) Figs, apricots and Dates

f) Lime, grapefruit and Lemon

g) Apple, mango, tomato, pear, avocado and papaya

h) Walnuts, pecans and almonds

1) Buckwheat, quinoa, oats, millet and brown rice

j) Brown-rice milk, almond milk

k) Coconut water and ground coconut

**Acid-forming foods are the following:**

a) Poultry, which include feathered game

b) Red meat, to include pork and venison

c) Commercially produced biscuits, breads and cakes

d) Processed breakfast cereals

e) Coffee, chocolate and tea

f) Cola, alcohol and diet cola

**Typical Alkaline Diet for a Day:**

**Breakfast**: Plain natural yogurt (Greek-style) with blanched almonds, fresh berries or Scrambled eggs, watercress/baby spinach, toast rye bread

**Lunch**: Wholegrain rye sandwich, buffalo mozzarella, alfalfa spouts and tomato or Quinoa/brown-rice salad, sliced avocado, diced chicken breast and rocket

**Snack**: Oat cakes or Hummus with vegetable sticks

**Supper**: Roasted butternut squash risotto, goat's cheese, parsley or Brown-rice sushi, miso soup, seaweed salad

## Chapter 5. Alkaline Diet Recipes for a Speedy Slim Down

A person can try alkaline diet if he or she wants to be energized or have a perk-up. This fast detoxification also helps to get start up your weight loss program. The way to a slimmer body is an effective digestive system. If you have difficulty shifting the pounds, or you feel bloated, it is crucial giving your system the needed break. When a person consumes food, his belly breaks down what he eats, systematically separating the nutrients from the waste, and eventually eliminates wastes through his bowel. Although this sounds so simple, it is actually a complex matter. This body system may be prevented in functioning at full capacity in many ways. Swallowing down your food quickly, poor meal choices, consuming too much alcohol can stress digestion, making it difficult to provide the body with the nutrients needed.

This is where the Alkaline Diet Recipes can be of help. Accordingly, the effect is immediate. Although the result may vary to every person, one can expect losing three pounds at least. Considering liquid diet in place of solid food for a short-term period can help in reducing burden of the digestive system, boosting nutrient intake in the process. The nutrients a person will be getting from smoothies and juices are numerous because the nutrients are in a pre-digested form already. This results to nutrients being released directly to the cells in order to perform their job effectively. This will deliver the rest that your hard working belly needed.

# Chapter 6. Juice Recipes

**The Early Riser**

This diet needs mixing of three squeezed oranges (fresh), five large strawberries, half banana, two tablespoons linseeds, one-tablespoon oats and a cup of water.

**Green Smoothie**

This requires mixing of half avocado, a cup of wilted kale, one large broccoli, juice of one orange, juice of one lime, a cup of spinach and water (400 ml).

**Tropical Beach**

Mix a cup of coconut water, pineapple chunks (one handful) and mango chunks (one handful)

**Glow You**

Mix palm full almonds, watercress (a handful), lettuce (a handful), juice of half lemon, chunks of melon, and strawberries (a handful)

**Green Goddess**

Mix half avocado, a handful of spinach, a handful of watercress, a chunk of cucumber, a pinch of sea salt, and cayenne pepper (sprinkled)

**Evening Beauty**

Mix unsweetened almond milk (one cup), one tablespoon chia seeds, raspberries (two handfuls), half apple, half avocado, and water (half a cup)

# Chapter 7. The Detox Plan

**First Day**

Upon rising: Drink warm lemony water

Breakfast: The Early Riser

Morning:  The Green smoothie

Lunch:  The Glowy You

Afternoon:  Nice Cup of miso soup

Dinner:  The Evening beauty

**Second Day**

Upon rising: Drink warm lemony water

Breakfast:  The Early Riser

Morning:  The Green Goddess

Lunch:  The Tropical Beach

Afternoon: a nice cup of miso soup

Dinner: The Evening Beauty

**Third Day**

Upon Rising: Drink warm lemony water

Breakfast: The Early Riser

Morning: The Green Smoothie

Lunch: The Glow You

Afternoon: a nice cup of miso soup

Dinner: The Evening Beauty

# Chapter 8. Losing Weight Through Alkaline Diet

Expert nutritionist highlighted ways in achieving a healthier weight permanently through exercise, proper diet and hydration through alkalizing. Accordingly, excess weight is commonly associated with several other health threats of fatigue, risk related to cardio-vascular disease and several other health concerns. Additionally, a critical distinction was observed on the subject of alkalinity and food intake that they are not only effective in losing weight, but also in building health and wellness. The purpose is on not only calorie restriction or self-depravity, but also more on re-balancing the pH and re-invigorating the body.

Nutrition experts stressed that the key in losing weight and health wellness is by increasing the consumption of green plant foods. Kale, parsley, wheatgrass, cucumbers, spinach, chard and watercress are at the top of the list to rebuild health. The above-mentioned plant foods have plenty of weight normalizing characteristics.

a) They are effective in reducing sugar intake because of their low sugar content.

b) They have high nutrients. These foods provide vitamins and minerals that are necessary for the body to function healthy and energized.

c) Being at raw state, these plant foods possess high level of electrons, which is helpful in facilitating energy flow inside the body.

d) These foods have good amount of magnesium necessary in the pumping of the heart and in eliminating toxins.

e) They contain chlorophyll, which is important building block of healthier red blood cells.

f) High level of fiber is found in them. Effective weight loss is also regarding the shifting of unwanted matters out of the body.

# Chapter 9. Alkaline Diet and Natural Bone Health

A medical expert relates the importance of improving the acid-alkaline balance in relation to bone health improvement. Accordingly, a person can acquire as many nutrients needed, do exercises and limit the toxins, but if the acid-alkaline balance is not aligned, it is possible to experience unnecessary bone loss. Therefore, alkaline diet is essential element of a person's natural bone health. However, most people nowadays, prefer meat, grains, processed foods, sugars and other acid-forming foods, but failed to balance them with alkaline-forming foods. Although human bodies can sustain infrequent acid load, the long-term acid accumulation may drain the available alkalizing reserves. If we are unable to neutralize acids, they may eventually affect our health wellness in many ways. This is also the reason of many health problems of people today, which include osteoporosis.

The general rule for alkaline diet recipes concentrates in whole foods such as root crops, vegetables and minimum level in nuts, fruits, whole grains, beans, seeds and spices. The diet is also inclined to alkalizing beverages including spring water and green or ginger root tea, and little amounts of meat, essential fats, fish, dairy and egg. Artificial and processed foods, white flour, caffeine and white sugar have to be eliminated as much as possible. You can dress your salads or cook your foods using high-quality fats (virgin olive oil, avocado oil, coconut oil).

# Chapter 10. Alkaline Diet Plan for a Day

The following is an alkaline diet recipe just to provide you with what to eat in order to achieve 80-percent of the diet. This diet does not concern restrictions on calories as well as elimination of some foods altogether.

Breakfast:

Veggie scramble: Use one to two eggs for every person, the eggs will be scrambled using green onion, some tomatoes, bell peppers and chopped bok choy. Match with ginger tea in a cup.

Snack:

One pear, a handful of toasted pumpkin seeds

Lunch:

a) Lentil soup with two cups of steamed vegetables (kale, broccoli, onions, carrots), Use olive oil as dressing for lightly steamed vegetables

b) 4 ounces hot or cold salmon (or tuna, tofu, chicken) served with 2-3 cups of mixed greens, cucumber, tomatoes, broccoli, carrots or other vegetables

Snack:

a) Eat Hard-boiled egg, you can slice them and sprinkled with few sea salt together with chopped parsley, celery, red bell pepper or carrot sticks.

 b) Handful of almonds

Dinner:

a) Take 4 ounces of chicken, fish or turkey with baked sweet potato or yam and mixed garden salad

b) Take pasta (made from rice, buckwheat, quinoa or amaranth) with bitter greens as toppings (broccoli, chopped zucchini, silver almonds or pine nuts, lemon juice, garlic, pepper and salt). Side dish: steamed zucchini with olive oil and garlic, add grating of fresh Parmesan

Seasonal fruits: (summer) get cherries and nectarines, melon, grapes, (winter) get baked apples, roasted pears

# Chapter 11. Alkaline Diet Recipes for Breakfast

The following recipes are alkaline diet suggestions for breakfast.

**Pancakes (Quinoa and Oat)**

This delicious alkaline American style pancakes are wheat free, dairy free, gluten and vegan free.

This recipe needs 80 grams ground quinoa, 40 grams ground, rolled oats, 10 grams ground flax seeds, 180 grams almond milk, 1 Dsp. Olive oil, a pinch of salt, a teaspoon almond essence, 1 Dsp. Tahini, 1 Dsp agave nectar (This recipe can be served using variety of toppings)

Preparation:
1. Grind, sieve quinoa, oats and flax seed
2. Mix ground flax seed, oats and quinoa in a bowl or blender with milk, agave and tahini paste. Mix until smooth
3. In a crepe or omelette pan, put few drops oil and heat up
4. Pour mixture (half a ladle) in the pan, cook for 30-seconds, turn the other side and cook again for 30 seconds, the pan should be kept at low heat, repeat for the rest of the mixture

5. Serve cooked pancakes with your choice of toppings, (wedge of lemon, agave nectar)

**Alkaline, Oat and Spelt Crepes**

This recipe requires 30 grams oats, 70 grams spelt flour, 180 ml almond or soy milk, 10 grams ground flax seeds, 2 Dsp live, zero-percent fat, plain soy, yogurt, 1 Dsp. tahini paste, 1 Dsp. agave nectar, a wedge of lemon, 1 Dsp olive oil

Preparation:

1. Grind and sieve oats and place in a blender with the flour
2. Add agave nectar, yogurt, tahini and milk, blend for few minutes 'till smooth
3. Pour and heat drops of oil in pan, maintain a medium heat
4. Using a ladle, pour enough mix covering the pan, cook for 12 – 15 seconds on one side. Use thin pallet knife and gently lift edges away
5. Slide pallet knife through center of pancake, gently lift, move inner edge to far side of pan, then turn knife towards pan gently, the pancake must role neatly into the pan.

**Breakfast Salad**

This is a light breakfast alternative. Energizing, low in carbohydrates and fat, full of alkaline nutrition. This salad is greatly serve with yeast free toast, avocado or nut spread.

Ingredients: 80 grams tender pea shoots, half avocado, ¼ cucumber, a stick of celery, ¼ red pepper, a handful mixed seeds, 2 sprigs fresh parsley, 2 sprigs dill, 1 teaspoon apple cider, 1 Dsp flax oil, juice of quarter lemon

Preparation:
1. Wash and prepare salad vegetables
2. Arrange vegetables in a plate
3. Sprinkle mixed seeds over the salad
4. Chop parsley finely
5. Mix the dressing, pour over salad
6. Garnish salad with chopped parsley
7. Season and serve

## Super Seed Breakfast Bars

Delicious bars that are great breakfast suggestion on the go. This is packed full of protein, slow the release of carbohydrates. Make great snack before and after workout.

Ingredients: 30 grams dates, 30 grams raisins, 30 grams ground almonds, 50 grams oats, 10 grams sun flower seeds, 10 grams pumpkin seeds, 10 grams gogis, 1 Dsp agave nectar, 1 tablespoon water, 30 grams flax seeds

Preparations:

1. Mix raisins, almonds, dates and oats in food processor, add the seeds after few seconds, finish the process by adding agave nectar, water until mixture became a firm dough
2. Lay baking parchment sheet, shape the mixture resembling a long bar through folding the parchment sheet along with the mixture. Shape it using spatula or rolling pin.
3. Raise parchment side, tip seeds on the top of bar, cover and set the seeds into the bar using a rolling pin.
4. Coat all the sides in the same manner.
5. Cut bars to equal pieces and chill

# Chapter 12. Alkaline Diet Recipes for Lunch

**Fondant Potatoes and Chilli Cabbage**

Tasty food combining vegetables with thyme and chilli, giving it a fresh bite, which will make you satisfied.

Ingredients: Half small savoy cabbage, 2 of baking sized potatoes, 1 red onion (chopped finely), 150 ml of vegetable stock, 3 Dsp Olive oil, 20 grams sun dried tomatoes, 1 Dsp Thyme

Preparation:

1. Preheat oven, 200c
2. Wash, peel potatoes, cut in half
3. Place pan on the hob, add 2 Dsp olive oil
4. When already hot, place potatoes face down, cook for a minute or until slightly brown
5. Turn potatoes over. Repeat the process.
6. If roasting tin is being used, add stock directly to the pan, season with thyme. Cook for 15 minutes.
7. Wash, shred cabbage. Steam for 8 minutes

8. Add remaining oil to a pan with finely chopped sun dried tomatoes, chilli and onions. Gently sweat for 4 minutes with lid on.

9. Serve potatoes and cabbage garnished with chilli and tomato mix.

**Steamed Winter Vegetable Medley**

A hearty, quick winter dish, packed full of alkaline energy and nutrition. The flavors make great low calorie food alternative to traditional Sunday roast.

Ingredients: 200 grams squash, 300 grams spouts, 200 grams leek, 200 grams carrot, 1 tablespoon per 15 ml extra virgin olive oil, 30 grams roasted chestnuts, 15 grams sun dried tomatoes, 3 grams finely chopped sage, 1 small onion (chopped finely), Salt and pepper

Preparation:
1. Wash, prepare vegetables
2. Slice the leeks, cut the squash, top, tail and cross sprouts
3. Dice onions, chestnuts and tomatoes finely
4. Chop sage finely
5. Steam the sprouts, leeks, squash for 8 minutes
6. Gently sweat tomatoes, onions, sage and chestnuts in pan using oil for 3 minutes, season and nicely serve over vegetables.

**Cream of Carrot and Pumpkin Soup**

This recipe is an alkaline soup filled with alkaline nutrition. It uses pumpkin and the soup is greatly served warm. Serves two if taken as main meal or serves four as starter.

This recipe needs 500 grams pumpkin, 500 grams carrot, 50 grams onions, 40 grams celery, 5 grams ginger, half teaspoon nutmeg, 120 ml almond milk and 400 ml stock soup.

Preparation:
1. Dice cut the pumpkin and the 230 grams of carrots, cut onions and celery in small pieces
2. Sweat all the veggies in the pan using a tablespoon olive oil in 4 to 5 minutes covered
3. After adding the hot stock, let it boil and cook further for 6 minutes
4. Juice the other carrots and the ginger; pour in a blender along with nutmeg
5. Spoon contents from the pan gradually into the blender and blend them until they are smooth
6. There is no need of straining the soup, but it can be served in a bowl with finishing of almond milk and seasoning

**Spring Vegetable Broth**

Simple and light spring broth, which only takes a few minutes preparation. It keeps the live, nutritional benefits of all the vegetables. Perfectly served for lunch as starters.

Ingredients: 150 grams spring onions, 1 small onion, 80 grams baby broccoli, 200 grams asparagus, 80 grams green beans, 4 basil leaves, 6 mint leaves, 400 ml vegetable stock, 1 per 5 ml olive oil

Preparation:
1. Chop small onion finely, put in pan with olive oil, sweat in three minutes at medium heat 'till soft
2. Pour vegetable stock in pan, bring to boil. Wash, chop vegetables, cut accordingly
3. Put vegetables into the boiling stock, simmer for four minutes. Remove from heat, add basil and mint, season and serve.

# Chapter 14. Alkaline Diet Recipes for Snacks

**Scotch Duck Eggs**

This recipe is an adaptation of a snack, which is low in fat. This is balanced with protein and complex carbohydrates, and is perfect for salads, buffets and snacks.

The recipe requires 4 duck eggs, 40 grams red onion, 250 grams of spouts, 50 grams ground sunflower, 20 grams sun dried tomatoes, 40 grams ground oats, 50 grams ground almonds, 5 grams fresh basil, 20 grams ground onion (dried) and a teaspoon of oregano

Preparation:

1. Wash the sprouts thoroughly and season lightly. Position the spouts on top shelf of the steamer.
2. Position the duck eggs in the bottom of the steamer. Steam spouts in four minutes and boil eggs in seven minutes if you choose the egg to be runny or ten minutes if well done.

3. Cool the eggs completely and remove the shell.

4. Chop onions and sun dried tomatoes finely. Slowly sweat them in a pan using 1 tsp olive oil together with oregano and seasoning.

5. Remove sprouts from streamer when done and drain. Place the drained sprout together with basil, bread crumbs and the sweat items from the pan in the processor. Blend the mixture until firm dough, but slightly moist.

6. Roll out right amount of dough for each egg. Mould the dough around the egg firmly, and coat them with breadcrumbs.

7. Fry the eggs with one tablespoon of olive oil at minimum heat for 3 to 4 minutes constantly turning them with thongs until reaching golden brown.

8. Plate the golden brown egg along with salad ready for serving.

## Apple & Rhubarb Crumble

High alkaline traditional English dessert. This alkaline diet recipe is best diabetic dessert.

This recipe needs 200 grams apples, 200 grams rhubarb, 40 grams raisins (optional for diabetic), 2 Dsp. xylitol (1 measure for crumble), 60 ml purified water, 200 grams whole, rolled oats, 200 grams sunflower seeds, 20 grams pumpkin seeds, 20 grams almonds, 2 Dsp virgin olive oil, 1 Dsp tahini, 1-teaspoon almond essence and 2 mixed teaspoon of nutmeg, cinnamon and mixed spice

Preparation:

1. Preheat oven, 200c
2. Peel and slice apples. Wash clean and slice rhubarb. Place in a pan with water, raisins, spice and 1 dsp xylatol.
3. Bring to a boil; simmer at medium heat in four minutes. Drain after cooking.
4. Blend almonds and seeds for few seconds. They have to be roughly chopped and not fine. Do the same with the oats.
5. Put all the dry ingredients, spice and xylitol in the mixing bowl. Add oil and tahini.

6. Mix the ingredients with tahini and oil establishing a crumble mixture.

7. Put the fruit in baking dish topped with the crumble mixture, and bake in 20 to 25 minutes.

8. Serve along with low-fat yogurt.

**Chewy Garlicky Toasts**

Ingredients: one (1) Red bell pepper, one (1) Jicama, six to 8 cloves of garlic, one (1) medium tomato, one-third (1/3) cup olive oil, one (1) teaspoon sea salt, Basil

Directions:

1. Slice the jicama not over 1/4" thick. Set aside.

2. Fine chop tomato using processor. Get the pulp by straining the juice.

3. Finely chop the garlic and the red bell pepper. You may want the moisture of the bell pepper to squeezed out because the vegetables have to be dry.

4. Stir the ingredients all together leave jicama.

5. Spoon enough amount of topping for each slice of jicama. Dehydrate them for about seven to ten hours just until chewy.

Notes:

a) Lots of oil is needed for this recipe.

b) The vegetables must be spread thinly.

**Sweet Potato Chips (Crispy Raw)**

Ingredients: one (1) large sweet potato, Sea salt, Olive oil

Directions:

1. Thinly slice sweet potato and place in a bowl.

2. Drizzle slices of sweet potato with olive oil. Sprinkle with right amount of sea salt.

3. Dehydrate chips using dehydrator at 115-degrees for twenty-four hours. The objective is for the chips to be crispy.

4. This makes two (2) dehydrator trays. Place in airtight container.

# Chapter 15. Alkaline Diet Recipes for Dinner

**Quick Chickpea Curry**

Ingredients:

Dish: 2 cups of broccoli & cauliflower (Chopped), 2 medium size tomatoes (chopped), 1 cup of dried chickpeas (need to soak overnight), 1 tablespoon olive oil

Sauce: 1 tablespoon curry powder, 1 medium size eggplant (chopeed), 1 clove garlic, a dash cayenne pepper, 1/2 cup water, 1 teaspoon cumin seeds, 1 teaspoon salt

Directions

The Sauce:

Blend at high-speed all the ingredients to puree

The Dish:

1. With oil, sauté chickpeas at med-high heat until golden.

2. Add the cauliflower, broccoli and tomatoes, continue cooking for ten minutes.

3. Get the sauce and pour from blender over mixture, then simmer for another ten minutes.

4. Serve and enjoy.

## Green Dragon Broccoli

Ingredients:

1 cup butter, almond

1 head kale (chopped)

2 cups broccoli (chopped)

1 bunch of dandelion leaves (remove from stem)

1 cup mint (well minced)

1 tablespoon butter, coconut

2 teaspoons hing

1 cup raisins

2 chillis, Thai dragon or jalapeno (chopped)

1 teaspoon tarragon

2 tablespoons lemongrass (well minced)

1 tbsp lime leaf

2 teaspoon salt

1 tablespoon ginger

1 cup water

Directions:

1. In a blender, blend mint, hing, peppers, ginger, raisins, tarragon, lemongrass, lime leaf, salt, almond butter, coconut butter and water until smooth.

2. Put wilted broccoli, dandelion greens, and kale with the marinade.

3. Apply liquid to vegetables very well. Pour the mixture to one larges casserole dish.

4. Put the dish in dehydrator in four hours. Set temperature to low.

5. Best served warm.

## Purple Pasta with Broccoli and Walnut Pesto

Ingredients:

Broccoli part–

One pack broccoli (tenderstem, about ten to fifteen stalks)

1/2 cup tamari

1/2 cup olive oil

1 tablespoon sea salt

Pasta part-

6 courgettes

2 cup raw beetroot

1 tablespoon sea salt

1/4 olive oil

Walnut pesto Part-

2 cup basil

1 cup walnuts

1/4 olive oil

2 teaspoon sea salt

2 tablespoon lemon juice

Directions:

1. Broccoli part-

2. Place broccoli in a bowl.

3. Add all the other ingredients. Marinade for two hours.

4. The bowl can also be placed in dehydrator at 115 degrees Fahrenheit to speed up wilting process.


Pasta part-

1. Juice beetroot, then transfer to bowl.

2. Cut tips of courgette (leave the skin).

3. Slice courgette into linguine type of strips.

4. Put courgette strips in the bowl with beetroot juice and add all other ingredients.

5. Set aside.


Walnut pesto part-

1. Pulse ingredients in food processor leaving mixture a bit chunky.


Assembling of all parts:

1. Remove courgette strips from beetroot juice mixture and drain.

2. In other bowl, gently mix walnut pesto with purple pasta.

3. Remove the broccoli and allow to drain.

4. Arrange broccoli in a plate.

5. Arrange pesto and purple pasta on the top of broccoli. For the sauce, blend 1/ 2 cup cashews with one cup of remaining beetroot marinade.

# Conclusion

Alkaline foods help in keeping the healthy body balanced. Most acidic diet leads to various health concerns such as poor circulation, weight gain, fatigue, heart ailments, memory loss, achy joints, constipation and other respiratory problems.

Getting the proper alkaline balance is essential to overall health wellness and effective weight loss. Understanding the benefits of Alkaline Diet Recipes lead to pH balance and increase of energy.

## Thank You Page

I want to personally thank you for reading my book. I hope you found information in this book useful and I would be very grateful if you could leave your honest review about this book. I certainly want to thank you in advance for doing this.

CPSIA information can be obtained
at www.ICGtesting.com
Printed in the USA
LVHW081542111121
703070LV00022B/630

9 781632 872739